Paleo

Power

Reclaim Your Health and Transform Your Body Through Paleo Diet

Jennifer Schwarz

Table Of Contents

Introduction — **3**

Chapter 1 — **8**
Why Paleo Diet — 8

Chapter 2 — **13**
What Is Paleo Diet, And How Does It Work? — 13

Chapter 3 — **16**
The Importance Of Developing Healthy Habits And Ways To Do So — 16

Chapter 4 — **25**
The Value Of Responsibility And How To Use It While Adopting A Paleo Diet — 25

Chapter 5 — **31**
Advice For Adopting A Paleo Diet — 31

Chapter 6 — **39**
The Paleo Diet Combines It All With Exercise — 39

Chapter 7 — **42**

Chapter 8 — **46**
Sample Recipes To Help You Get Started On The Paleo Diet. — 46

Conclusion — **50**

Introduction

Nowadays, it seems like someone is attempting to persuade us that their method of improving our health is the best wherever we turn. The world might seem to be an incredible place full of wonderous technologies enabling us to lose weight quickly between fad diets, supplements, and items that promise to perform miracles. And making a decision may be daunting and challenging, especially as you learn the harsh reality behind many of these choices. Scams exist, chemicals and hormones may be changed in the body and have devastating side effects, and miracle-working items can have long-term negative repercussions.

So who can we rely on to start living a healthy lifestyle?

There is an easy solution: Nature.

There is a delicate natural equilibrium present in nature. The obvious outcomes will be damaging to us if we deviate away from natural methods and replace things like healthy nutrition and exercise with drugs and famine. We were made to thrive on a plentiful diet abundant in certain nutrients, such as good fats, vitamins, and minerals.

The paleo diet may help in this situation. The notion of eating only foods that our Paleolithic predecessors ingested was first proposed in the 1970s by Walter Voegtlin, and it has since gained enormous popularity. The concept is that we restrict many starchy items and fatty meats and stick to meals that are nutrient-rich and ideal for maintaining the body and gastrointestinal system as happily as possible when we cease consuming foods introduced during the period when hunting and gathering slowed down into farming. He believed it would be a successful strategy to persuade people today to eat more healthfully.

Voegtlin pioneered his profession, and his studies influenced others to come to their own conclusions regarding food. Another medical professional thought our bodies were designed for this kind of nutrition. Specifically, to consume the same foods that our ancestors, who were hunter-gatherers, could get while on the go. Lean meats, fruits, vegetables, nuts, and seeds are easy for us to digest naturally. In reality, they are beneficial to humans. Foods like grains, maize (really a grain), and dairy products ingested in large quantities may cause the body numerous problems. These foods became widely and economically accessible to humans via farming. There are several different sensitivities to this kind of marketed and everyday staple food, including lactose intolerance, gluten sensitivity, and others. A few of them are also quite starchy, which might make it challenging to lose weight.

The Paleo diet is excellent for those who want to lose a few pounds, but it is also a significant lifetime commitment. It's not only about looking nice; it's also about feeling wonderful and making beneficial decisions. Knowing that the things we choose to consume are harming our bodies may be incredibly problematic. There will always be a weight on our shoulders when we consume items that we know are terrible for us, even if we aren't consciously aware of that particular damage. We typically grasp what is good for us and what is bad for us instinctually.

Although decreasing weight isn't the Paleo diet's main objective, it is a huge advantage. The likelihood that you are currently experiencing physical effects from the Standard American Diet, also known as the SAD diet, due to the appalling lack of nutrients in typical meals served when consuming processed, pre-packaged meals are very high. We'll discuss how harmful processed meals are in a later chapter. So giving up these unhealthy items and deciding to adopt a Paleo diet are both major game changers. You'll feel better than you have in a long time in both your body and mind! All because of a simple switch.

Going Paleo isn't some fad diet where you have to buy a journal and count every calorie you eat to know if you are doing it right (although to be honest, there is some benefit to some journaling if you want to hold yourself accountable to the choices you are making.) If you are overeating and not getting enough exercise to burn the calories you eat, then calorie counting can benefit you. However, suppose you are doing Paleo correctly. In that case, many individuals might go too far with that strategy and fail to consider the nutrients they could be missing when they adhere to fad diets. The paleo diet is very different. You don't need to pull out a large, intricate map to plot your course. You just need to take a step back and consider how our predecessors managed to maintain excellent physical health via natural means. Also, we can!

Look no further if adopting a Paleo diet is your

correct decision. This manual will assist you in beginning the delightful path of eating foods as they were intended to be eaten. Stop with the sad crap now! Then let's get going!

Chapter 1

Why Paleo Diet

Why go Paleo, you may be thinking? What makes it different from, say, keto? Also vegan? Also Atkins?

The solution is elegant in its simplicity. The Paleo diet is distinct because it is more of a way of thinking than a specific cuisine. It offers a fresh perspective on life and a great lens through which to choose foods. Stating, "I can only eat this many carbohydrates today because of my diet," isn't as positive as stating, "I can have a complete dinner, and it will be great!"

This is because, as opposed to the ketogenic diet, where you are compelled to restrict your carbohydrate intake to a hazardous level to the point that your body is essentially in starvation mode, and you lose weight rapidly, you are only channeling your food choices so that they are all of the healthy sort. You don't want to consume junk food containing undeclared sugars, excessive amounts of salt, and preservatives. You should consume meals already abundant in the nutrients our bodies need to flourish. You want a natural diet!

The Paleo diet was created for this reason. Because it wasn't laden with carcinogens and other unknown dangers, the guy who invented it hoped to persuade everyone to eat as our Paleolithic predecessors did. It was a clean method to receive your nourishment, enabling you to withstand the weather and thrive. If the Paleo diet was so beneficial, some could question why individuals from that period didn't live longer. That has an easy solution. They endured very risky living situations. They did not have modern medicine like we do. Since they had to have strong immune systems to withstand the conditions, they could naturally combat illnesses that may have killed us.

What type of society would we live in now if we had access to the technologies we have created today?

The Paleo diet is a healthy method to maintain a balanced body, a sharp and alert mind, and the flexibility and skill we would have needed in survival conditions thousands of years ago.

The fact that this diet isn't as important nowadays is a

blessing. What would it be like to see someone who was reared on a diet of fast food and prepared meals attempt to outrun a wild animal? Or even better, use their resourcefulness and simple equipment to battle and destroy it? Or even someone who followed a strict ketogenic diet to lose weight rapidly. Without the right quantity of carbohydrates in their system, they might end up passing out. Do you believe that those who abuse their bodies out of convenience would prevail in a life-or-death scenario? No way!

The idea behind the Paleo diet is straightforward. You want to perform to the best of your abilities. The body is a fuel-powered machine by nature. The quality of the fuel we put in our automobiles is directly related to what we put into our bodies. That is a typical gasoline form if we routinely consume fruits, vegetables, and meats. But if we load up on junk food, preservatives, high fructose corn syrup, processed items that are already packed, and fast food, we may as well put diesel in an engine meant to operate on unleaded. We must work harder to take better care of our engines to prevent breakdowns! Switching to a Paleo diet is a fantastic way to eliminate the things harming your body, even if it's not obvious. Consuming unhealthy meals often impacts us in ways we are unaware of until it is too late to make a difference. For instance, consuming meals that are heavy in fat and salt may start to harm your arteries. When your doctor informs you that you need to lower your cholesterol, it may come as a major surprise to you since you don't feel it is occurring. In the worst situation, you have a heart attack before you realize anything is amiss. It is easy to see why heart disease is one of the major causes of death in the United States.

Thankfully, adopting a Paleo diet is easy. It is simple and obvious why this is such a fantastic option. It consists of lean meals and good fats that benefit the heart rather than harm it, as opposed to clogging arteries with fatty red meats, fat, and salt. And when it comes to making decisions that impact your body, that should always be the goal. Not hurting is what you want to do. All of your actions will come back to haunt you. If not now, as you become older, your body truly begins to suffer the consequences of your decisions.

Fortunately, it's never too late to make adjustments that can benefit your body and mind and enhance your health! Even though making any kind of lifestyle change, particularly one as fundamental as changing one's eating habits, might be intimidating at times, the reality remains that we want to improve our lives, health, and world.

Our health and our lives depend on it, and there's no reason not to start Paleo immediately if that's the chosen route! Some of the fundamentals will be covered in the next chapter. Put your thinking hat on and start figuring out how to incorporate Paleo into your life.

Chapter 2

What Is Paleo Diet, And How Does It Work?

This is most likely the question that is now consuming your thoughts. What exactly does adopting a Paleo diet entail? What should you eat, and what shouldn't you consume? And why is it okay to do certain things but not others? Dairy wasn't around when people lived in caves. Or was it?

Simply put, the Paleo diet differs from other diets because it emphasizes whole foods without adding flavors or salt. They consumed what was around them, went on foot to hunt for meat, and collected berries, nuts, and seeds. They did not often have fixed lifestyles. They were always on the go because they had to follow the herd. Paleo is more than a diet. It is a way of life. Foods that are Paleo-approved and a sedentary lifestyle just won't have the results you want them to have. You should remain active and receive a sufficient quantity of daily exercise. Now and again, you should increase your heart rate to ensure you exercise your body to the utmost.

That does not imply that you should proceed with caution. Consult your doctor about the appropriate workouts if you have limitations. Paleolithic people didn't spend their days lazing in caves, playing on their phones, or watching television. They went outside, roamed about, and survived by eating what the environment gave them. Therefore, it isn't true to state that the Paleo diet will magically solve your weight problems since it won't. Like any diet, it functions best with active living and other healthy practices.

Let's dive into the specifics of how this diet works now. Here is a short list of the meals you should include in your paleo diet. These foods consist of:

- Fatty meats. Consider the animals you could kill, especially those that consume grass, like deer. Game meat.
- Vegetables of every kind.
- Various kinds of fruits.
- Fish, especially salmon. Everything you know is rich in omega-3 fatty acids.
- Seeds, nuts, and seed- and nut-derived oils.

It seems very easy, doesn't it? Let's now discuss the kinds of meals you should avoid consuming. They consist of the following:

- Lentils, peas, beans, etc. No sort of legumes.
- Dairy.
- Salt.
- Potatoes contain starches.
- Swift meal.
- Processed sugars.
- Fatty meal.
- Prepared meals.
- Grains. Yes, bread is included in this.

That's pretty much all there is to it. It seems so basic, right? That's correct; it is! Going Paleo has that as its main benefit and ultimate goal. Simplify the meals you consume to simplify your life. Remove anything with additives that are challenging for our bodies to assimilate so that we may advance more quickly without anything unneeded, obscuring our thinking and blocking our arteries. That's how simple it is.

Chapter 3

The Importance Of Developing Healthy Habits And Ways To Do So

Having the resolve to change anything in our lives is difficult. In addition to being motivated to act, we must possess the skills and abilities to keep our objectives at the forefront of our minds and take the baby steps required to get there. It is quite easy to become inactive, lose focus on the actions that move us ahead, and revert to poor behaviors that will set us back if we aren't always trying to improve our lives and ourselves.

Although the Paleo diet is straightforward, it will not be effective for you if you lack discipline. There will still be advantages, of course, but there is no sense in reading any further if you can't learn to say no to your vices and start making changes in your life that you can keep up with. Unless you want to learn how to alter it, that is!

There are many excellent resources available to assist you in developing a healthier lifestyle and changing your behaviors. We all have amazing potential to develop, and if we can consistently see the pot of gold at the end of the rainbow, it will be much simpler to keep moving in that direction.

Because making a significant overhaul of our lives may be highly intimidating and challenging, many individuals quit before they even start. The habits we have are difficult to break. We develop emotional attachments to our way of life and certain items that cause our bodies to produce endorphins, such as meals with a high sugar or fat content or other substances that are addictive for similar reasons.

However, we do not have to depend on unhealthy meals and allow ourselves to make poor decisions. Holding ourselves responsible for developing healthier habits is essential to better managing our lives and growing into the strongest versions of ourselves possible.

We lead. When we reach a particular age in adulthood and have to make decisions regarding our health based on how we manage our time and money, we can't put the responsibility on anyone else. Some things in this world are beyond our power to influence. We can let things like that go. However, we can't let go of what is within our reach. We simply cannot allow ourselves to deteriorate because it is the simpler course of action to give up before we have even started or established genuine, lasting new habits to replace the old ones.

Most of the time, perseverance and patience are the keys to creating new habits. We must be clear about what we want, keep our sights on the goal, and simply go for it without hesitation or apology. What if your family or friends don't want to join you on your paleo journey? Who cares if the people around you continue to make the same poor decisions you pledged not to? That does not entitle you to abandon your objective.

Those folks are free to make their own decisions, which is ideal. You have a goal that you know would improve your life, but you can't let peer pressure influence you or allow yourself to relapse into a vice and justify it by saying it's what everyone else is doing. Take responsibility for your decisions and treat yourself with respect.

You may live the paleo lifestyle alone or with the help of others around you if you wish to consume wholesome, unprocessed meals. You need to act ethically in both scenarios. Make decisions for yourself. For the benefit of yourself. The likelihood that your new lifestyle won't last increases if you merely do it to lose weight, look good, or join a trend. You could subsequently be reminded of the item you previously attempted but abandoned since it will be another brief period in your life. It might be hard to remember the things you don't accomplish to the best of your abilities. When we are reminded, we may experience guilt. We feel guilty for not caring for our bodies better than we should have. And those emotions may deepen into sadness or sentiments of self-pity, sometimes resulting in even worse decisions.

Prevent that! Make an effort to create and follow healthy decision-making practices. You will feel stressed if you don't, since we should be able to stand up and say we gave it our all. Because the decisions we make are significant and because we are significant as well, we should be proud that even when we encountered a challenge or gave in to temptation and fell off the wagon, we were able to get back on. We must feel proud of ourselves for sticking to our decisions and living in excellent health, eating wholesome meals that feed our bodies.

But it's easier said than done, isn't it? Habits are challenging. They have nervous systems. They are mental. Roadblocks that keep us from really caring about ourselves, our decisions, and our effects on the world around us will undoubtedly appear and cause your plan to fall apart.

Attempts to adopt a healthy lifestyle. So how can you get around such obstacles? What can we do to recognize them and put a stop to them?

First, it is helpful to pause and consider what we are doing for our own benefit versus what we are doing to harm ourselves. Make a list, if necessary. Consider every aspect thoroughly. Do you get enough shut-eye at night? Do you get enough liquids? Do you work out every day? Are you a weekly cardio user? Are you maintaining a clean, sanitary living environment? Are you emphasizing your mental health and removing toxic connections from your life so they aren't clogging it up and making you question your value?

If you want to start making better decisions for yourself and staying with them, it is crucial to address all those issues. Creating healthy habits will become very difficult if you continually weigh yourself down with negativity and don't prioritize your mind, body, and health.

If necessary, consider why you aren't doing what you want. Has someone in your life advised you not to worry about yourself? Do you consider yourself deserving of a better life? Don't lose hope if you think a deeper-rooted problem may prevent you from making adjustments in your life that may benefit you. For people who wish to sift through the reasons they don't want to make better personal decisions or don't feel good enough, there are many accessible tools.

Some of these possibilities include seeking therapy, consulting with a life coach, or just engaging in certain meditations that will direct your attention toward the problem and help you discover a solution. The best way to start making life-altering changes that will last is to understand who you are. Equally crucial is holding oneself responsible for those decisions. You can't simply let something go if it has significant value. You need to put up a fight to hang onto it and be in command of giving that crucial item top priority in your life. Nobody else will do it for you; most people will make it worse since they are unmotivated.

Everyone has their preferences and requirements, and they can even be pressing for something from you. When attempting to achieve anything, all of those things might be distracting. No matter who may be in the room objecting or criticizing you or just living in their habits without realizing how alluring those vices could be, you have to have the courage to know that the decisions you make are important enough to you to follow through with.

Developing new habits might take a week to a month, depending on how determined you are to continue the new routine and how often you can practice it. The easiest method to start a new habit is to prioritize it and stay with it daily around the same time.

Time. Humans like routines; these ritualistic actions come naturally to us since we need them to survive. It will be much simpler for you to maintain this habit if you can arrange your meal plans so that you eat at around the same time each day.

Taking your time if going paleo is completely new to you is recommended. One habit at a time should be the first to modify. For instance, if you depend on refined sweets, consider weaning yourself off them first and getting used to the little adjustment before making the bigger one. In this manner, you may transfer more easily and maintain your determination. It's crucial to stay on course!

Therefore, you should correct yourself as quickly as possible if you forget a day or eat something you know you shouldn't. Otherwise, instead of reinforcing the new habit you're attempting to form, you can simply revert to the old one. Stop blaming yourself, becoming angry, or getting upset about it. Recognize that it did happen and that you are human and may improve. Then improve! It's not difficult; you just need to make a decision and stick with it through thick and thin.

The most crucial aspect of developing a habit is remembering that it takes time. Don't consider how challenging it may be to struggle for a prolonged time to refrain from eating items you know you shouldn't. Consider the days you were successful, then concentrate on one day at a time. That is the most efficient technique to achieve your goal. Avoid completing everything at once or being distracted by

the big picture. Simply consider the day-to-day
decisions you must make and strive to make the
correct ones!

Chapter 4

The Value Of Responsibility And How To Use It While Adopting A Paleo Diet

Building new habits might be difficult, as was described in the previous chapter, but it is always possible! However, it may be challenging, and we often need structure to keep us on track. It's one thing to form a habit; it's quite another to maintain it. When creating your paleo lifestyle, you will want to take great care to get back on the horse when you stray and think, "What will one time hurt? I have been doing so well!" since you have been doing so well. Sure, a one-time slip-up can be a nice indulgence, and any unhealthy lifestyle decisions you make in moderation may be less harmful than if you made those bad decisions all the time. However, you do not want to get into the habit of making excuses for yourself when you do something that you know is contrary to a very specific goal or lifestyle you have in mind for yourself.

If you allow yourself to indulge once, you may wish to indulge again later, and whatever discipline and self-control you have managed to maintain will soon be gone. Maintaining a new lifestyle may be difficult, and if you aren't prepared to put in the necessary effort, you will never achieve your goals.

You are, however, that much closer to making it so simple that you do it without even missing the way you used to live if you are prepared to keep yourself responsible, whether by writing about your paleo journey or by developing charts outlining your problems and success stories. The days of overindulging in unhealthy habits will seem almost like a nightmare. It's comparable to how someone who has stopped smoking and hasn't touched a cigarette in around ten years might sometimes comment that they can't believe they ever did it in the first place since it feels like a lifetime ago. Going paleo is similar in this regard. If

If you are ready to put in the effort to make this work for you, you will one day reflect on the unhealthy decisions you made and be shocked and bewildered by the thoughts that were running through your head at the time.

Journaling is a powerful technique. Writing down your successes and your challenges can help you come up with a strategy for how to handle them in the future. By journaling your journey, you may learn more about what can make you want meals that you know are terrible for you. You may therefore avoid stressful situations and concentrate on ensuring that you are in circumstances that enable you to make the healthiest decisions for yourself.

For instance, if you are seeking something processed, you may use the tried-and-true bait-and-switch technique: consider the item you are craving and compare it to a healthy option. Perhaps you could try a leaner beef burger instead of your preferred fast food establishment's cheeseburger. You can simply locate bread substitutes or make lettuce wraps. The bun is scarcely noticeable.

There are several varieties of bread substitutes. Flax seeds make excellent bread substitutes. More gluten-free choices could be suitable for you. Simply ensure you read the labels of the things you consume carefully before eating them to avoid making a mistake that can confuse your body.

Speaking with friends, family, and coworkers about your diet is a wonderful substitute for keeping a diary. It may also be helpful to keep coworkers informed. You should let anybody know that you have altered your lifestyle before they ask you out to a location where it will be difficult for you to get a nutritious dinner. In this manner, if they see you reaching for anything you know you shouldn't rely on a paleo diet, they will have the chance to inquire whether it is appropriate for you to eat that item and your future diet goals.

Making simple charts or checklists to keep oneself on track is an alternative if writing things down and reaching out to your community to start a support group isn't enough. You may simply hang them on your refrigerator door to remind yourself to try to achieve your daily objectives. For instance, you may have a line that reads, "Paleo Meat," "Paleo Vegetables," or "Paleo Fruits," with a box next to it for a checkmark and perhaps a yes or no box.

If you tick the "no" option, you may want to add a line asking, "Why?" or any other phrase encouraging you to do better tomorrow.

Because it might be quite easy to dissuade yourself from ever taking up the diet to try again, it is crucial not to punish yourself too harshly for slacking off. You don't want to traumatize yourself before you've even had a chance to achieve. Many of us have a negative mentality that suggests we can't accomplish the goals we set, and the first time we mess up, it appears to confirm this.

We get upset and saddened when our thoughts support this ridiculous notion, and it seems we keep doing so with more and more mistakes. There is no reason not to live an authentic paleo lifestyle if we can forgive ourselves, move on, rapidly fix our errors, and return to where we began so we may keep moving the right way. Even when our brains work against us and tell us we have no control, it is still within our grasp. We need to disprove it, particularly to ourselves.

We won't appreciate the force of responsibility unless we know our power. We will stop living the helpless lifestyle that eventually causes us to decay and feel miserable all the time and start making the decisions that allow us to feel powerful and confident while also knowing that we are capable of achieving the objectives that we set out to achieve if we stop constantly making excuses for ourselves and instead concentrate on ways that we can improve and do things in a better way. Nothing is more satisfying than that.

Chapter 5

Advice For Adopting A Paleo Diet

You can do several things to make the paleo diet work better for you than simply following the straightforward advice of avoiding specific foods and hoping for the best. For instance, did you realize that eggs fit within the paleo diet? And you'll get a nice protein boost if you consume the whole egg. Either egg yolks or whites are just OK. Additionally, these are both foods that our prehistoric predecessors would have consumed.

Going paleo is simpler if you do it with a friend or partner, like most things in life. More power to you if you have a partner, spouse, or friend eager to alter their lifestyle alongside you and work on developing novel and intriguing meals that are enjoyable and filling. If you want to recruit someone else to do it with you, go ahead! Having a companion while going through this huge lifestyle adjustment might make it a lot easier. Even better, consider giving them a copy of this book as a reference to keep you both on the same page. Those puns, oh my.

Now, remember that there may be such a thing as too much fruit juice since juicing fruits removes the fiber from the fruit, leaving you with a lot of natural sugar in one location most of the time. If you need anything other than water or tea, it would be best to look at methods to make it naturally rather than juicing, even if it is still tasty and has some vitamins to its credit. It may do wonders to just leave some pulp in your juice. So try that out. Fruit may be consumed on this diet even though it contains natural sugars. Just be careful not to overdo it, and everything should work well. They may be an excellent method to gradually wean yourself off packaged meals and snacks, which are extremely harmful and make you feel regretful rather than satisfied.

It's also a good idea to discover alternatives for what you want rather than using a lot of self-control to keep yourself from giving in to temptations instead of concentrating on what you wish you had and want. There are excellent methods to substitute items, such as the suggestion in the preceding sentence to swap out sugary sweets with fruit-based ones.

Some individuals adhere to fairly rigid paleo diets, eating only foods they believe the cavemen would have consumed. This might severely restrict your creative freedom in the kitchen. You can have a lot of fun in the kitchen with the options you do have, so try not to let yourself become trapped in a box like that. Imagine what magnificent dinners the Paleolithic man might have prepared if he had had access to modern conveniences and the same supplies. He probably did have some originality in his cuisine to some extent. Being able to do this practically serves as a survival mechanism.

Speaking of what our ancestors may have consumed, it is doubtful that their food included pesticides or was raised on a diet containing growth hormones. Try your best to remove any items that contain unnecessary chemicals if you can, get organic products. Healthy eating and avoiding items known to cause cancer go hand in hand. Ultimately, we don't want to endure pain in our later years due to something that might have been easily prevented. Isn't achieving health in the first place meant to do that? It's a good idea to think about becoming organic to reduce the chemicals we ingest in our bodies that might lead to problems later in life.

Crock pots may be a fantastic purchase for anybody considering adopting a paleo diet. They make it simple to combine meat and veggies to create a flavorful and delectable dish. It's simple, reasonably priced, and excellent! Additionally, by using a crock pot to prepare your food rather than baking or frying it throughout the summer, you may avoid generating extra heat in the home.

Purchasing soups is a smart move if you're following the paleo diet. Soups are simple to make, keep well, and may be stored and thawed later. Stews function similarly and provide excellent backups when you're exhausted. You can avoid going to fast food places if you remember that you have stew or soup that you can unthaw and then just heat up if you get home late and are tempted to eat something quick and on the run. A quick supper! Having it as a backup is fantastic because it prevents you from overindulging in foods you don't want to consume. You may indulge your body indulgently and yet enjoy the same comfort. Because you're spending less on food, it could be more convenient.

Speaking of cooking, it may be helpful to prepare

your meals in advance and large quantities throughout the week or weekend so you don't run out of time later and find yourself tempted to go for something quick. Even if it may appear difficult to prepare every meal every single day, that may simply be

Resolved by preparing food in advance. Even better, you can heat frozen meals to extend their shelf life. Similar to your homemade microwave meals, but without salt and other unhealthful ingredients and preservatives. There are several approaches to making self-catering simple and practical. Finding the time to complete it is all that is required.

Trying to consume as much of the animal as you physically can without becoming ill is something you could find objectionable, but that might benefit you in the long run. This suggests you should try organ meats. You don't want to reject some of the animal's most nutritious components and waste them. That's not what our forefathers would have done! Numerous health advantages may be obtained by eating organ meats; as far as taste is concerned, you may even come to like them. You can't learn until you try!

Keep yourself hydrated throughout this time, don't

forget. Water consumption is essential. Your muscles and cells benefit, and your body functions as efficiently as possible. Drink more often if you exercise vigorously or if the weather is hot and you notice that you are sweating for any other reason. Ensuring you are maintaining your whole body, not just the food-related areas, is crucial. The paleo guy would have taken care to drink plenty of water and exercise as much as possible. His way of life required it. No one was an exception. No waste, either. It is a fantastic lifestyle to aspire to.

Reading food labels to ensure you aren't unintentionally ingesting something you don't want to consume is one aspect of becoming paleo that might be challenging. Manufacturers may smuggle all sorts of stuff into their goods. If you believe something to be chicken, it may not be. Who knows what more elements have been added? Salt and other preservatives are often added to increase the shelf life of foods. Being friends with local farmers who rear their animals on precise, nutritious diets and offer them to clients in season may thus be a smart option. Because everything an animal eats becomes a part of them and subsequently becomes a part of us, it is preferable to ingest animals with a healthy diet.

Hormones should not be consumed indirectly. They should not be taken lightly since they have previously been connected to several severe diseases.

Growing your garden might be another fulfilling endeavor you like. Access to fresh fruits and veggies may save you a ton of money since you won't have to worry about what has been handled or sprayed on your food or how it was treated before it reached you. Make sure you study the safest methods for gardening so you can meet any requirements it may have. They might be a little finicky but are generally rewarding and can produce much! If you're inventive enough, you can grow plants in the city. You may learn how to achieve it by using a variety of resources.

One of the most crucial things to keep in mind is to have your sights set on the goal. Consider what motivated you to start the paleo diet, and always keep that inspiration near.

Your brain. If necessary, put it in writing and keep it someplace you can see it often. Simply visualize your objective and remind yourself of the reasons you must keep doing the actions necessary to reach it. Everything you do will ultimately have an impact on you. The decisions you make are issues you must deal with. Possibly not now but later. Additionally, if you choose poorly today out of convenience, the same conveniences could not be available to you later. And it is simply a plain, regrettable law of life.

However, everything eventually finds a balance, and as long as you keep working toward your objectives and are honest with yourself when you make mistakes, everything will return to normal. You shouldn't berate yourself for having a cheat day. Remember that it's an indulgence and not something you should become accustomed to. Remember that you have a better strategy for your next meal, a plan that will enable you to permanently attain your objectives. Never return to your paleo diet; remember why you chose it!

Chapter 6

The Paleo Diet Combines It All With Exercise

The one thing about our Paleolithic predecessors that we can say with absolute certainty is that they were active. To live in a harsh environment and ensure that the people they loved the most could eat and flourish, they had no alternative but to exercise their bodies and build their muscles. No one of us would be where we are now without that commitment. We would go extinct as a species.

Thankfully, our forebears had the motivation to relocate. They were motivated to live. And we still have that drive now. We need to discover new methods to harness that energy. We no longer stroll through woodlands for food as a vital survival strategy. We visit the supermarket. We maneuver through concrete slums. If we give it any thought, we visit the gym. However, we aren't chasing after animals and killing them to feed our families. Most of the time, we are not in constant motion like our forefathers. And it may cause serious issues for our bodies.

The paleo way of living entails more than simply dieting. We must make sure that our bodies are being used. Making a decision not to sit around all day watching TV or hibernating. Going paleo in our meals is unlikely to have the greatest impact on our health if we aren't attempting to be active. Just remember that although eating healthier may help you lose weight, it won't do much to tone your muscles if you have a precise idea of what it means for your body to go paleo. Only exercise can do that.

Members of our Paleolithic ancestors could have engaged in several forms of exercise. The amount of running, lifting, hauling, crouching, and climbing they likely did is not insignificant. In a struggle for existence, all of those things happen naturally. Even swimming is a possibility for them to have done.

In addition. Just consider how long it would have taken to follow a herd to a new area while walking around. It may be quite difficult to keep in shape and lead as healthy a lifestyle as possible if we aren't making use of the fact that our bodies are designed for movement.

Fortunately, maintaining your physical fitness is simple. Walk outside each day, for instance. Stretch your muscles. Every few days, let yourself 20 minutes of cardio. Starting and maintaining an exercise regimen is the toughest part, but you may utilize the guidance provided in the chapters on developing habits to start moving in the right direction! Nothing can prevent you from constructing a better life by taking the necessary actions. You just need to be concerned enough to make and keep the commitment!

Chapter 7

Meal Planning For Paleo Diet

One of the most crucial things you can do to manage your money and diet is to schedule your meals. This is because having a strategy to follow may be beneficial. You can immediately go to your meal plan, get your items, prepare your meals, and divide them out rather than feeling rushed and confused about what to do for supper since you haven't yet planned anything. This may assist you in staying on course and avoiding becoming sidetracked by fast fixes and simple solutions that are ultimately highly damaging.

Some individuals find it difficult to organize their dining out. They tend to be impulsive, and their appetites fluctuate, so they could find it difficult to sit down and carefully consider the meals they want to include in their meal plan. A meal plan, however, is not designed to restrict your freedom. Using it properly should improve your performance, provide more alternatives, and help you save time and money. You must have many more creative options if you are saving money, don't you think? To make meal planning simple and enjoyable, remember that you don't have to set any restrictions. Consider including in your meal plan the things that you genuinely really like eating. In this manner, attempting a new cuisine or recipe every day won't overwhelm you. The thought of it can be overpowering. It takes a lot of effort! But if you want to make sure you consider familiar, reliable items you genuinely feel at ease with, then simply keep them in mind as you plan your meals.

But if you're adventurous and want to try something new, you may readily check cookbooks and other sources for recipes. Perhaps you could save a fresh dinner on one day each week.

Experience. It can be a day when you intend to eat leftovers from the previous evening so you would have something to fall back on if you don't like what you had prepared. However, it was generally advised not to waste food, particularly in Paleolithic times.

Checking what foods you already have is a smart idea before organizing your meals for the week so that nothing you have purchased will go to waste. Being mindful of what you use and when you use, it may be a wonderful tactic if you want to ensure that your new diet motivates you to live a waste-free lifestyle. Don't throw away your fresh fruits and veggies. Check the expiration dates of your fruits and veggies to determine which ones are most likely to go bad earliest. Use them while they are still fresh. Make consuming those meals a priority!

Additionally, while arranging meals, don't be hesitant to utilize leftovers. Using them creatively may enable you to save money and add a humorous touch to your meals for the week. Making a side dish that can be used in various ways, such as a side dish one day and as a topping the next, ensures that your food will last a long time and reduces the likelihood that you will waste anything you purchase. By practicing portion control, you may prevent yourself from overindulging in meals simply because you know they are better for you than other options would have been.

One last advice for meal planning is to prepare for the possibility that you won't feel like cooking at some point. Be prepared for it. Perhaps you could prepare a soup or stew and freeze it to be ready when you need it. Or maybe you can prepare something twice as much at the beginning of the week so you will have it later when you feel worn out and don't feel like cooking.

Naturally, you can still toss ingredients in a slow cooker on days like those and let it do the bulk of the job. It is a nice backup plan for days when cooking simply doesn't seem attractive. In any case, be sure to be reasonable while making your meal plan so that you can stick to it and feel good about it. Because you have lofty objectives, don't go overboard. Work within your current limitations and gradually push yourself to go beyond. And be practical in your approach! Otherwise, you can get stressed out and think you've failed when you really need to take things a bit more slowly and have just overloaded yourself.

All of this is significant, but beating yourself up if you make a decision that you later regret is not worthwhile. Work hard the next time to avoid making that decision instead! By doing this, you'll have a fresh slate at every meal, giving you plenty of chances to choose foods that are as healthy as they can be.

Chapter 8

Sample Recipes To Help You Get Started On The Paleo Diet.

Breakfast recipe: Burritos Paleo breakfast

Ingredients

2 Paleo tortillas
2 Eggs
1 Red bell pepper
½ yellow onion
Pepper to taste

Directions

Cut the yellow onion and red bell pepper into dice. Warm up the paleo tortillas in any way you choose. You can reheat them in the microwave or a pan over medium-low heat for a few seconds on each side. Till the required level of heating is reached, flip regularly.

Cooking spray should be heated over medium heat in a medium skillet. Together, cook the yellow onion and diced bell peppers until the onions are translucent and the bell peppers are tender. About 4 minutes after the eggs are cracked into the pan, stir them until they are well cooked. Place in a tortilla, season to taste with salt and pepper, and serve hot.

Lunch Recipe: Paleo turkey lettuce wraps

Ingredients

8 slices of deli turkey meat
2 big pieces of lettuce for the wrap
Salt and pepper to taste
1 sliced avocado
Sliced or chopped tomato
Mayo to taste
Fresh basil sprigs to taste

Directions

The more lettuce leaves you can spread out, the better. Cover the lettuce with the mayo and basil sprigs. The avocado is then added. Place the deli slices on the lettuce, sprinkle with the tomato, and then wrap them up. Serve right away and enjoy chilled.

Dinner recipe: Paleo Slow Cooker Chicken Recipe

Ingredients

3 cups of vegetable stock
2 boneless, skinless chicken breasts
Pepper to taste

Directions

Use the ingredients of your choice to season the chicken. Simple pepper will do for this dish. After that, add the chicken breasts to the slow cooker with the vegetable stock, ensuring the liquid covers the chicken breast. You may change as necessary. Turn on the slow cooker and use the high setting to simmer until done. Depending on your slow cooker, this should take about 2.5 hours.

Dessert recipe: Amazing Peanut Butter and Banana Smoothie with Cacao Nibs

Ingredients

2 Frozen bananas

2 cups of almond milk

2 teaspoons of raw peanut butter

1 tablespoon Cacao nibs

Directions

First, whirl your blender on high while adding the frozen bananas. Although it should be done in the blender once finished, this may also be done in a food processor. Add the cacao nibs and raw peanut butter after the almond milk. Blend for 30 seconds until the smoothie is the consistency you want. If you want a thicker consistency, add ice cubes, which shouldn't be processed in a food processor. When the smoothie has reached the correct consistency, pour it into a glass and serve immediately.

Conclusion

The thought of altering their way of life might be intimidating for many individuals. In all honesty, it truly is. To make it work, a lot of effort and commitment is required. But if you are prepared to work hard and follow through on the decisions you know will improve your life, there is no stopping you! Adopting a Paleo diet may first appear difficult. Still, in actuality, it may start to seem quite simple if we truly concentrate on making the decisions we are certain will assist in bringing us to a better life.

With the excellent and straightforward paleo diet, you could discover a whole new outlook on life. Accepting that a bad meal that formerly had us in its grasp was a vice and one we honestly no longer want is tremendously gratifying.

Every so often, falling off the wagon is normal. It might be challenging to make several changes at once, so it's crucial to remember that we're not simply adopting a paleo diet for aesthetic reasons. We do it to improve our lives, our bodies' efficiency, and the quality of our thoughts. The endorphins we obtain from exercising and eating well will make it practically hard to get sad and may result in a beautiful attitude shift. And it is significant.

The most important aspect of altering your way of life is always to remember to forgive yourself. Undoubtedly, we all make bad decisions. We all make decisions we later regret. It may be upsetting to learn that sometimes we treat our bodies and self with less regard than others. But don't allow your shame and remorse to stop you from grabbing your desired life. Even if you keep telling yourself otherwise, you do deserve it. Work on the problems you recognize as problematic.

And recognize the ways they prevent you from pursuing the life you want. After dealing with them, you may go forward.

Our diets are a very significant and individual matter. Many of us have strong attachments to our meals because they significantly influence who we are. We form bonds with food and create memories around it, so it may be frightening and depressing when we stray from the comfort foods and favorites that we have become used to enjoying with the people we care about. But keep in mind that we are not abandoning the things we cherish. To live and love even longer than we planned, we love ourselves enough to make good decisions.

Additionally, brand-new routines may be created around your new likes and diet. You may discuss them with family and friends and be confident that you are taking the necessary steps to spend as much time as possible with the people you care about.

You are responsible for deciding what success means to you. Never allow someone else to complete it for you. Going paleo will give you more self-awareness and confidence than ever. Before reaching the summit, you must confront yourself and genuinely push past any little issue holding you back. And if you're not ready to look in the mirror, all you can truly hope for is to run into circumstances that won't depress you.

Don't let life happen to you; don't be that person. Create a life for yourself by taking control of it. It was intended to be that way. Did they wait for animals to come to them during the Paleolithic era? No way! They went outside and located the herd, which they followed until they had acquired all they needed.

Follow their example. They got up and started living their lives. No matter how difficult it looked, they first determined their requirements, then went out and did what they needed to do to live. We are still here on Earth due to that desire, which they instilled in every one of us. We continue to experience daily life. Now live that life to the fullest while respecting their memory.

Although adopting a Paleo diet won't solve all of life's problems, it will undoubtedly make you more resilient to whatever may come your way. In addition to making you look and feel fantastic, eating well and losing weight will ensure you always give your all to anything you do. And we, as well as our forefathers, may be quite proud of that. Give it your all while you're out there, then! There is no excuse for not being your best self, so do it now.

About The Author

Jennifer Schwarz is the owner and creator of kenvi Consulting, which offers various services to help you be as successful as possible. She's passionate about helping people get healthy and happy. Jennifer loves yoga, music, and teaching people how to be their best selves. She's also the writer behind Pure Yoga: Mastering the healing art for Health and Peacefulness, Organize your life: A most efficient method to organize your life, The untapped gold mine of diet, weight loss, and many more.

She is not a nutritionist or trained chef, just a determined mom who searched high and low for a way of eating that would reduce inflammation and allow her to live a happy and healthy life.

Jennifer lives in Dallas, Texas, with her husband and two beautiful children.

Other Books By Jennifer Schwarz

350 Low Carb Cookbook: Quick and Delicious Low Carb Recipes Can Help You Lose Weight Effortlessly

DIETING AND WEIGHT LOSS: 5 Unexpected Dieting and Weight Loss Tips

Coconut Oil: Discover The Amazing Benefits of Coconut Oil From Skin Care, Hair Moisturizing, Weight Loss, Digestive Aid, Immune System Booster, & More........

CBD HEMP OIL: Use Hemp Oil To Look Better and Feel Better

Pure Yoga: Mastering The Healing Art For Health And Peacefulness

TOP KETOGENIC DIET: The Quickest & Easiest Way To weight loss

14 Days: To A Better KETOGENIC, DIET

A Guide To KETO, DIETING At Any Age: A Perfect Guide to Losing Weight, Boost Your Energy and Eating Healthy

The Untapped Gold Mine Of DIET, WEIGHT LOSS : That Virtually No One Knows About

Delicious And Healthy Diabetic Recipes: Over 500 Tasty And Healthy Recipes To Take Care Of Your Well-Being Without Sacrificing

Super Health For Super Kids: Parenting Guides For Picky Eating And Stronger Immune System

Respect All Life: Tasty Vegetarian Food And Cooking

Healthy Juicing: Exploring the Science, Nutrition, and Impact of Juicing on Your Health and Well-being

One Last Thing…

Dear Reader,

I hope you enjoyed reading this book and found it to be valuable for your needs. As an author, it means a lot to me when readers take the time to leave a review on Amazon. Your feedback not only helps me improve my writing but also helps potential readers decide if this book is right for them.

If you have a few minutes to spare, I would greatly appreciate it if you could leave a review on Amazon. Your honest opinion can help other readers make informed decisions and can make a real difference in the success of this book.

To leave a review, simply click the link below and follow the instructions. It only takes a few moments, and I will personally read each and every review to gain insight into what worked for you and what didn't. Your input can help me create even better content for my readers.

Review link:

https://www.amazon.com/review/create-review?&as
in=B0BCHM3VK2

Thank you for your time and support. It truly means a
lot to me.

Best regards,

Jennifer Schwarz